PELVIC FLOOR PHYSICAL THERAPY SERIES:
PREGNANCY BOOK

YOUR BEST PREGNANCY EVER

NINE HEALTHY HABITS TO EMPOWER YOU IN PREGNANCY, BIRTH, AND RECOVERY

D1279855

BY

JEN TORBORG, PT, DPT

First Edition: June 2018

ISBN-13: 978-1720824480
ISBN-10: 1720824487

Pregnancy Red Flags

If something ever feels wrong, trust that feeling and talk to your health care provider right away, especially if you're experiencing any of the following:

   *changes in vision, blurred vision, dizziness

   *vaginal bleeding or leaking fluid from the vagina

   *sudden or severe swelling

   *difficulty breathing, shortness of breath that is worsening

   *severe or persistent vomiting

   *severe or long-lasting headaches

   *unusual or severe cramping in lower abdomen

   *fever or chills

   *discomfort, pain, or burning with urination

   *have thoughts of harming yourself or your baby

FREE BONUS

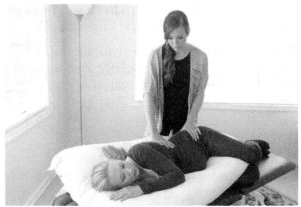

Photo credit: Kelsey Lindsey

Hi! I'm excited to share my knowledge with you on this amazing journey of yours.

To help you keep track of the healthy habits you may consider forming during pregnancy, I created **Your Best Pregnancy Checklist** to help you reach your goals.

To access the pdf, just enter the following URL: *jentorborg.com/Pregnancy-Checklist*

Check list also included at the end of the book

Enjoy!

Jen Torborg, PT, DPT (Doctor of Physical Therapy)

EUCALYPTUS LEAVES

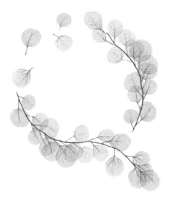

Artwork by Ana-Maria Cosma

Eucalyptus leaves represent healing and protection.
The eucalyptus tree is known for nurturing
— a plant for your pregnancy journey.

CONTENTS

INTRODUCTION

So you want this to be your best pregnancy ever?

I want that for you too!

My goal in writing this book is to reach pregnant women near and far who have questions about what they should be doing for a healthy pregnancy, a better birth experience, and a smoother recovery. I hope that you will take away practical advice and a feeling of empowerment during this time of your life.

I'm a physical therapist (PT) who specializes in pelvic floor physical therapy. I have my Certificate of Achievement in Pelvic Health Physical Therapy (CAPP-Pelvic) and Certificate of Achievement in Pregnancy / Postpartum Physical Therapy (CAPP-OB) from the American Physical Therapy Association.

I live, work, and play in a rural area of northern Wisconsin near Lake Superior. I know all too well from friends and clients that it can be hard to get to appointments for preventive care or treatment due to insurance, financial reasons, scheduling, location, transportation, etc. It would be awesome if every woman could have a pelvic floor PT on her team during her pre/postnatal care—someone who can help you through your questions about what is right for you as it pertains to how your body is moving and changing. Although I fully believe in an individual approach to each person's care and that no book, blog, or YouTube video will ever fully replace that, there needs to be more quality resources available, especially simple, easy-to-digest ones.

This book is written from the perspective of a PT whose passion is sharing straightforward, effective advice. My intention here is not to include an exhaustive list on everything you need to know during pregnancy. I aim to relate some very practical advice you can start using in your daily life right now. *(Plenty of healthy habits are included in this book regardless of pregnancy status, age, and gender.)*

Do this for me: While reading this book, imagine your best friend is a pelvic floor PT. That means she (or he, or they) knows all about what's up down there (bladder, bowel, sexual function). She can help answer the questions you don't want to ask your mother. You're sitting down together, and she's about to share with you what she wishes you knew.

There are quotes throughout this book from other healthcare professionals to compliment the message I seek to bring you. Most quotes are originals given specifically for this book. Links to more information from these providers are in the resources appendix.

*This book does use cisnormative language. I am a white, heterosexual, able-bodied, cis woman and this is where I feel comfortable speaking from due to my own life experiences, although I do want to acknowledge that sex anatomy and gender are different. There is relevant information for all pregnant people in this book, but the subject matter and terminology is aimed at cis women.

Here are two quotes to start us off. Keep in mind these words as you read this book and encounter other advice along the way:

> "It can be scary and discouraging to watch your body change and grow in ways you've never known. Sleep is slight, you are aching in places you didn't know could ache, and your whole self is getting soft and round: something society has told us to avoid our whole lives. Know this, though, you are an absolutely stunning woman made even more beautiful by a healthy, growing belly. Own it. You are courageously giving up your body to a life you don't know yet. Your body—the one you've nurtured and abused, the one you've loved and criticized—is building an *entire* human being. It's magical! *You* are magical. But this can be hard and overwhelming. Try to give yourself credit and grace for all you're doing when you don't feel like you're doing enough because you are a resilient goddess capable of unimaginable wonders."

> — Kelsey Lindsey, LPC-IT

> "Pregnancy is magical time in a woman's life, which allows her to connect to and inhabit her body in a whole new way— maybe even for the first time. An incredible wealth of healing, empowerment, and connection to Source (literally) resides in the pelvic bowl. Become keenly aware of the changes in your pelvis and womb space during pregnancy, birth, and in the transition into mamahood. This awareness will allow you to tap into the great power which resides within you at the base of your spine, at your core."

> — Casie Danenhauer, DPT, RYT

Throughout this book I hope to empower you in your ability to listen to your body and see what it needs. I'll provide advice about what you should be listening and looking for.

Your body was made to do this. You are a strong, resilient, powerful woman. Take this time to trust in yourself and gain confidence to having your best pregnancy ever!

XO
Jen

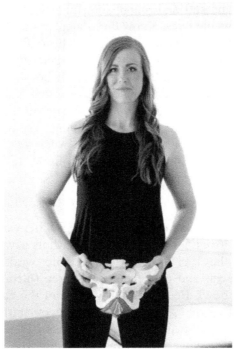

Photo credit: Kelsey Lindsey

HABIT 1:
EMBRACE YOUR BREATHING

Let's start this book by taking a nice, deep breath!

No, seriously, one of the first habits I hope you're able to adopt is to use breathing strategies to your advantage. Breathing can be used to calm your nervous system and relax your body. It can be a helpful strategy in the way you respond to stress and things you can't control. It can be a gateway to stay more present in this sometimes crazy life. Learning how to breathe for relaxation can help your physical and mental health as well as your baby's health. *It can even help improve your laboring and birthing experience.*

Find a moment to breathe in deeply through your nose, and then gently let it go through your mouth. You can breathe in whatever way you feel most comfortable (just nose or just mouth if you prefer) and whatever length of breath you feel is most natural.

If you don't have any reference for what feels best to you, consider:

- Breathe in (through nose) for a count of 1, 2, 3
- Breathe out (through mouth): 1, 2, 3, 4

As your baby grows inside you and pushes up against your diaphragm, you may notice it's harder to take deep breaths. Your diaphragm is your breathing muscle located like a dome along the bottom of your rib cage, the top muscle in your core. During this time, it's helpful to keep a comfortable amount of rib expansion when you take a breath in. Rest one hand on your chest and another on your belly. While breathing in (inhaling), you should feel your belly rise and *ribs expand out to the sides*. Keep your neck and shoulders relaxed. As you breathe out (exhale), you should feel your belly fall as the air pressure leaves your body. This type of breathing should not be forced. It should be a nice, gentle movement like waves going in and out. Diaphragm breathing can help strengthen and relax the pelvic floor muscles by engaging and lengthening them with pressure changes inside your body.

Find ways to fit this relaxation breath in throughout your day:

- between tasks

- in your response to stress, anger, anxiety, or worry

- during commercials

- before or after a meal

- upon waking or before bed

- as you arrive at a stoplight or are stuck in traffic or if your version of traffic is stopping for a deer or tractor

You may also want to check out other forms of relaxation breathing (all can be searched for on Youtube):

- Alternate nostril breathing

- Box breathing

- Extra exhale

- Extra inhale

- Breath of fire

It's beneficial to pay attention to your breath with movement.

Breathing during times of exertion or effort can help you achieve a healthy pregnancy. Clench your fists together as hard as you can. Now exhale. Did you realize you were holding your breath? Frequently throughout the day, as we are physically or mentally exerting ourselves, many of us tend to hold our breath.

This increases the pressure inside our body. Breath-holding done frequently (or intensely with straining) can sometimes have negative consequences on the body. Long-term breath-holding could contribute to pressure system issues such as urine leakage, prolapse, pain, blood pressure issues, hernias, and abdominal separation.

Personally, minimizing my breath-holding has made such a difference in decreasing the back pain I used to experience.

Checking to make sure you're not breath-holding while concentrating really hard or while exerting yourself physically—lifting the dog food bag, bending to pick something up, or even rising from sit to stand—is a good habit to have.

When exerting yourself, let that air go. Exhale on the movement.

For a better birthing experience, here are my general recommendations with breathing during labor and birthing:

- Don't hold your breath.
- Ideally, try to exhale with any pushing.

Recap of Embracing Your Breath:

1. Are you aware of your current breathing habits or style?

2. Do you hold your breath frequently? When?

3. Can you replace those breath holds with an exhale?

4. How do you envision fitting in more relaxation breaths throughout your day?

HABIT 2:
KNOW YOUR PELVIC FLOOR

How many of you know your pelvic floor? I mean, how many of us actually know what I'm talking about when I say that? What muscles I'm referring to? What's their purpose? Can you feel them contract, relax, and lengthen?

Prior to going into pelvic floor PT, even with a background in anatomy and physiology, I had only a vague sense of what the pelvic floor was. I knew some of the other parts: bladder to urethra, uterus to vagina, rectum to anus—but the muscles? Sadly, no. I have a distant memory of reading an article in Cosmopolitan when I was young. It was the first time I heard of Kegels. All I can remember was squeeze those muscles = Kegels.

Did I have any clue what I was doing? No, not really. Oftentimes in my practice, I find that the reason pelvic floor dysfunction occurs is due to a lack of knowledge about this area. We don't typically see it, touch it, and talk about it like other areas of our body. If the only advice you've ever gotten is Kegels, this chapter is sure to give you many more quality instructions.

"Kegels are technically the contract-and-lift part of a pelvic floor exercise. Did you know there's more to a pelvic floor exercise than simply contracting? As we move through the day, pelvic floor muscles are contracting (and lifting up) and relaxing at various levels with breath and movement. One should also be able to actively contract and then relax. And believe it or not, the muscles should also be able to bulge (not the same as straining) to allow for urine and bowel voiding."

—Tracy Sher, MPT, CSCS

Maybe you've heard of Kegels before. Maybe you haven't. Let's dive into the actual anatomy of what we're referring to—your pelvic floor muscles. We'll discuss them in detail to improve your awareness and understanding.

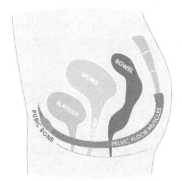

www.burrelleducation.com
©Burrell Education 2014

Your pelvic floor muscles are made up of multiple individual muscles connecting to different points and located at different depths. In general, they are the muscles that go from your pubic bone in the front to your tailbone in the back and your sit bones (ischial tuberosities) side to side. These muscles wrap around all three openings: urethra, vagina, and anus. They make more of a bowl than a floor.

The goal of your pelvic floor is to keep your pelvic organs (bladder, uterus, and rectum) supported up and inside you and to keep your urine, stool, and gas in until you're ready to go. Your pelvic organs are intertwined with your sexual experience, and they help with stability and movement.

They are pretty important, yet often overlooked. Most of us have a hard time knowing exactly where these muscles are because we don't see or touch them the way we do with most other muscles. You can watch your bicep contract when you're at the gym or picking up around the house. You're able to get feedback to your brain with your vision and touch (out in public!) in a very quick, easy, and socially acceptable way. Unfortunately, most of us have a more abstract image of our pelvic floor muscles and sometimes feel there's a stigma that keeps us from talking openly about them.

Let's demystify these muscles and how they work.

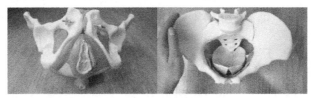

Don't think of your pelvic floor muscles as an isolated group. Your pelvic floor muscles work as part of a system that is sometimes called the core, although I use that term loosely because it means so many different things to different people and professions. If I use the word *core*, I'm referring to the core of your body like the core of an apple or the core of the earth—the deepest, innermost part.

So, in that sense, other muscles worth considering are the transversus abdominus muscle, kind of like your own inner corset. This muscle is deep to all the other abdominal muscles and wraps from the front to the back—usually felt best just inside your pelvic bones in the front. This muscle typically contracts and relaxes with the pelvic floor muscles. Sometimes while you're pregnant, it feels like you're hugging the baby when you engage the transverse abs. Other muscles involved are the multifidus (muscle group along the spine) and the diaphragm (your breathing muscle), the roof of the core, which really relates all the way back up to how you breathe.

Why are we talking about all of this?

Studies show that women who perform pelvic floor exercises correctly during pregnancy may have:

- decreased labor and birthing times

- less likelihood of urine leakage during pregnancy and postpartum

- faster postpartum recovery
- less chance of tearing or need for episiotomy

Learning about this part of your body now may help you stay strong not only during pregnancy and postpartum, but also throughout the rest of your life. *Feeling empowered about where and how these muscles work is a healthy habit for your best pregnancy, birth, and recovery.*

Pelvic Floor Exercises

Why is there such a huge chapter of this book dedicated to pelvic floor exercises when most other pregnancy books and blogs have only a few sentences on them? It's because studies show an estimated 50 percent of women perform these exercises incorrectly.

It should be noted that Kegels in the traditional sense (squeeze, squeeze, squeeze) are not necessarily appropriate for everyone. Your pelvic floor muscles should have the ability to do what all muscles do—not only contract, but also relax and lengthen. It's important that your pelvic floor work in coordination with the rest of your body.

> "To kegel or not to kegel? During pregnancy it is important to keep your core as strong as possible, to balance out the change of gravity due to the baby as well as the joint laxity from the change in hormones. The pelvic floor is part of the core, so it is essential to keep the length tension and strength as optimal as possible. But if someone has any overactive or pain conditions, then they typically need to release and lengthen the muscles before they strengthen, which requires more deep breathing techniques and manual therapy."

> —Amy Stein, DPT, BCB-PMD

Common mistakes made while trying to do pelvic floor exercises:

1. **Squeezing different muscles than you intend to** such as butt cheeks, inner thighs, and upper abs. Those muscles aren't going to help hold back the urine or gas.

2. **Overusing your upper abs or obliques** may increase the pressure inside your abdomen and onto your pelvic floor. If done

repetitively or intensely, it could lead to (or worsen) diastasis recti abdominus (DRA), pain, prolapse, or leakage.

3. **Squeezing too hard or all the time**. If you squeeze your absolute max all the time, the muscles are going to begin holding tension and have difficulty relaxing. We don't constantly keep our other muscles tensioned all the time, nor do we repeat max reps of the same exercise over and over without rest. It's important to have a balance of contracting and relaxing while being able to vary the intensity of your squeeze.

4. **Breath-holding.** When I had my first internal exam to see if I was performing my pelvic floor muscle exercises correctly, I thought I was going to nail it since I hadn't been experiencing any pelvic floor problems and was able to stop the flow of urine as needed (all those practiced Kegels since the day of reading Cosmo!), but guess what? I was holding my breath every single time, and it was very difficult for me to contract my pelvic floor without doing so. Breath-holding puts increased pressure on your pelvic floor, and it is not a sustainable or healthy practice to only be able to squeeze with breath holds. I now have better quality contractions and ability to relax because I breathe when I squeeze.

5. **Only being able to squeeze or relax with a certain tilt of your pelvis or in a specific position**. Maybe you learned to do pelvic floor exercises when someone told you to flatten your back against the floor, or you've only ever practiced them in sitting. We move through many positions during our day-to-day routines, and it's key to be able to utilize these muscles in all postures and positions.

Are you convinced of the importance of improving your awareness of your pelvic floor and the power it is capable of?

When you first begin learning pelvic floor exercises, I recommend timing with your breath to tap into the natural pressure changes that occur while you're breathing in and out.

The concept of a pressure relationship between the diaphragm and the pelvic floor (and much more!) is taught as Piston Science by Julie Wiebe, PT. She has been integrating these concepts into movement, function, and all forms of fitness (CrossFit, running, etc.) from the start. She is an advocate for empowering women to keep pursuing fitness in the midst of pelvic health and pain issues. She deserves a ton of credit for creating and giving a voice to this integrative approach which is now widely used by pelvic floor PTs. Check out her YouTube videos and online programs for more information. Links are located in the resources appendix.

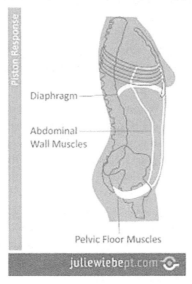

Here are some cues used to help women begin connecting with their pelvic floor muscles:

Let's use the exhale (decreased pressure inside the body) to help you contract and the inhale (increased pressure inside the body) to help you relax your pelvic floor muscles, and then an exhale again to help you lengthen your pelvic floor muscles.

Try your best to not hold your breath or engage other muscles. *Remember, no one should be able to see you squeezing!*

Contraction

In a comfortable position, take a breath in and relax, then on an exhale, imagine the following:

- You're in a crowded elevator, and right behind you is your celebrity dream crush. Try to stop from passing gas without squeezing your butt cheeks.

- Pretend you're on the toilet. Try to stop the flow of urine.

- Visualize where your pubic bone and tailbone are. Try to bring them up and in together.

- Picture both sit bones (ischial tuberosities) and pull them up and in together.

- Visualize your vaginal opening and your anus. Close those openings and lift up and into your body.

- Sometimes simply exhaling through your mouth as though you were blowing out through a straw will actually engage your pelvic floor automatically.

- Imagine a red kidney bean at your vaginal opening. On your exhale, close and lift the kidney bean into your body (note that your butt cheeks won't help that kidney bean lift in), and then don't forget to inhale to relax and let that kidney bean go.

  o Thanks to Julie Wiebe for the bean cue!

Which cue worked best for you? What visual felt like it helped engage your pelvic floor without overusing other areas or wanting to hold your breath? Could you also feel a gentle contraction inside your pelvic bones in your lower abdomen (transverse abs)? They're supposed to work together.

From now on, when you hear *contract your pelvic floor*, try to remember the cue that worked best for you.

"Shortened pelvic floor muscles have a difficult time contracting and going through their full range of motion. […] Relaxing the muscles between exercises is as important as the exercises themselves. Your muscles won't function with optimal strength unless you learn how to relax them."

—Amy Stein, DPT, BCB-PMD

Relaxation

The majority of the time, your pelvic floor muscles should be resting. If you're sitting at your desk concentrating hard on a task, in heavy traffic, or in a heated conversation, take note of the tension throughout your body, including your pelvic floor, and work to let that tension go. Relax.

Some cues that are helpful:

- On the inhale, feel the pressure inside your core increase, and let it lengthen your pelvic floor back to a relaxed position.

- Imagine your vagina as a flower opening or butter melting.

- "Let the bean go"

Lengthen

It's important that we don't stop with the contract-and-relax routine, but also consider what all muscles in our body should be capable of—lengthening.

Being able to lengthen your pelvic floor muscles, especially during bowel movements, urination, and childbirth, can be extremely helpful.

You should be able to lengthen the pelvic floor muscles without holding your breath or straining.

Cues for a technique called "belly big, belly hard" can help lengthen the pelvic floor:

- Take a nice breath in, and gently let your belly expand.

- Continue to keep your belly expanded with use of your abdominal muscles. Engage "belly big, belly hard" as you transition to an exhale.

- As you exhale with "belly big, belly hard," gently lengthen your pelvic floor past its resting position.

Not sure if you're getting it?

To locate the pelvic floor muscles:

*Toilet test for checking your contractions. Next time you have to urinate, try to stop the flow. Can you do it? This gives you some feedback on whether or not you're activating your pelvic floor. *Please don't actually practice these exercises on the toilet, though.* Only test here maybe once a month or so. We want to have a nice, constant flow when urinating and not to disrupt it or cut off too early. Rest in the restroom!

*Towel test. Roll up a small towel and sit on it from your pubic bone to tailbone. Perform your pelvic floor exercises. You should be able to feel a slight lift off the towel on contraction. Relax back to the towel, and then slightly bulge into the towel on lengthening the pelvic floor muscles.

*Watch your pelvic floor muscles. Depending on the size of your belly at this point, grab a mirror and separate your labia (the folds) so that you can visualize the vaginal opening, then practice your breathing pelvic floor exercises:

- inhale, relax

- exhale, contract

- inhale, relax

- exhale, lengthen

What do you see? Can you see a gentle close (lift up and in)? Also, if you bear down, can you see the pelvic floor relax and lengthen? *Do you see anything bulge out past the opening? This may be a prolapse and is worth mentioning to your health care provider.*

*Feel your pelvic floor muscles. If you're open to this option of connecting with your body, *I highly recommend it.* Find a comfortable place, maybe lying down or in the shower. Imagine the vaginal opening as a clock and 12:00 is toward the clitoris and 6:00 is towards the anus. With a clean (perhaps lubricated) finger, enter your vagina to your first knuckle pressing down to the 6:00 position. Try to contract, relax, and lengthen to see if what you think you're doing matches what you feel. Then enter the finger a little further onto the 3:00 or 9:00 position, and try the exercise again. You should feel a lifting or contraction of the pelvic floor muscles as you "lift the bean," and you should feel the muscles relax back down as you "let the bean go." You should also feel the muscles lengthen as you bear down.

Still unsure and want more feedback?

I recommend asking a professional specializing in the pelvic floor to give you feedback on your ability to contract, relax, and lengthen to be sure it's matching with what you're perceiving. Consider seeing a pelvic floor PT for detailed assessment. Links to find a PT near you are located in the Resources appendix.

Now that you know how to perform pelvic floor exercises, when and how often should you do them?

Pelvic Floor Exercises with Your Breath

I recommend combining your goal of taking time to breathe with your goal of getting in tune with your pelvic floor muscles.

A few times throughout the day when you take breaths to clear your mind or transition to the next task, add in your pelvic floor contract-and-relax routine.

Inhale = let your lungs fill with air = abdominal pressure increase = relax tummy/pelvic floor ("let the bean go").

Exhale = air leaves your lungs = decrease pressure in your abdomen = activate pelvic floor ("gently pick up the bean").

On a regular basis, you don't always need to practice the lengthen portion, but it's good to check in every now and then, and make sure you have the ability to do so. Bowel movements are a great time to check that you're lengthening properly without breath-holding or straining!

Once you arrive at 35 weeks of pregnancy, increase daily focus on the lengthening of your pelvic floor during exhale as a way to prep you for labor and childbirth. The goal of this is to decrease chances of tearing by improving your ability to relax and push without breath-holding.

Mix it up. Learn to vary the intensity of your squeezes. Be able to contract anywhere from your max to 50 percent effort to even less than 25 percent effort.

Just like you have the ability to contract your bicep at different intensities on demand and for different functional goals (picking up a pen versus picking up your kid), you want to have the ability to vary your pelvic floor muscle recruitment.

A few times throughout your day, add in pelvic floor exercises with your relaxation breathing.

Begin to feel confident doing this in a variety of positions: lying down, sitting, standing, on your hands and knees, and in a deep squat. Now let's add them to movement.

Pelvic Floor Exercises While Moving

We don't live our whole life in predictable patterns or staying in one place, so don't stop with only performing pelvic floor exercises in a static position.

Begin by adding pelvic floor exercises to a portion of your current exercise program. (Don't currently exercise? We will cover that in Chapter 4.)

During each exercise movement, recognize where the most exertion or effort is required, and start by timing your exhale there to optimize the pressure in your body.

Example: If I was doing a lifting motion overhead (usually the lifting-up part is the hardest for me), I would blow out as I lift overhead. Depending on the length of your movement, you might breathe out for the whole movement or exhale for one part and inhale for the other.

Then as you get the timing of the breath down, add in your pelvic floor contraction to the exhale and your pelvic floor relaxation to the inhale.

Here's the sequence (one after the other within microseconds to transform into a nice, smooth movement):

Take a breath in and relax the pelvic floor, then...
Breathe out + contract "gently pick up the bean" + movement.
Then inhale and relax "let the bean go" between reps.

No holding your breath and no clenching that pelvic floor nonstop throughout your entire exercise routine.

It's not that you have to do this with every single exercise all the time, but adding it in to a few of your exercises intentionally should carry over to the rest of your movements with time.

It's also not that you need to or should breathe out with every single rep or exertion, but it's a good place to begin if this concept is new to you.

Over time, the goal is that this will become automatic to your body. The way learning something new, like learning an instrument or a new job, first requires a lot of mental concentration, but with practice and intention, it gets smoother and easier.

Ways to add it to exercise:

*Seated marching: Practice breathing out and engaging your pelvic floor as you lift one leg up in a march, and then set it back down. Alternate legs back and forth. At first, do one exhale-and-squeeze combination per leg movement. Inhale and relax between leg movements. The goal is to really feel the pelvic floor engage right before the leg moves and continue to feel it throughout the motion.

*Reaching overhead: Practice breathing out and engaging your pelvic floor as you raise your arms overhead, and then bring them back down. Inhale and relax between arm raises. The goal is to feel the pelvic floor engage right before you move your arms and continue to feel it throughout the motion. You can do this in any position: lying down, sitting, standing, or on your hands and knees. You can add weights to your hands if no weight feels easy.

*Standing squats: Hang on to a countertop or railing if this is new to you. Start with the exhale-and-squeeze combination throughout the whole movement. As your squat gets deeper or you add weights to your squats, you may choose to inhale and relax on the way down and exhale and squeeze on the way up.

Add this to whatever form of exercises you are already participating in. Once you get the hang of breathing and coordinating your pelvic floor it should start to become automatic.

Now maybe you're only engaging in exercise programs a few times a week. How do you add this to your daily life?

Real-Life, Daily Pelvic Floor Awareness

Use the same concept just described with exercises on movements you perform throughout the day that require physical exertion:

- Sit to stand from a chair—blow out and squeeze just before and while you stand up
- Bending down to pick something up
- Coughing or sneezing
- Lifting
- Reaching into a cupboard
- Getting in and out of bed (good one to remember early postpartum)

- Getting in and out of the car

- You'll want to use this with picking up your baby & lifting a carseat

What about things that are not rep-based—things that are part of your daily movements and longer than a simple moment of exertion, yet still require physical strength such as walking, running, stairs, biking, and swimming?

Here is where I tell you to ditch the idea of trying to time out each breath + squeeze + move and inhale + relax + rest but still maintain the general concept.

As you're going for a walk, you want the pelvic floor to cycle through contracting and relaxing. You don't want it to be clenching on for dear life the entire time, but you also don't want to ignore it and not have the ability to call upon it if needed.

Try this:

When going for a walk, pick a time or distance away that you'll do a self-check on your posture, breath, and pelvic floor.

So when I pass that beautiful tree up ahead, I ask myself:

1. How's my posture? Are my ribs stacked over my pelvis?

2. How's my breath? Am I taking nice, full breaths, or am I breathing really shallow and labored?

3. How's my pelvic floor? Can I feel it contracting and relaxing naturally?

Maintaining and Advancing Your Pelvic Floor Exercises

The goal of learning this now may feel overwhelming at first. If these concepts and body parts are new to you, it may take more mental strength than physical strength to master.

Remember, the goal is that the more you practice this concept, it will just become part of your normal coordination and movement patterns that fit easily into your daily life.

The easiest and probably most natural way to engage your pelvic floor is with your breath coordination. But just like we don't live in one posture or position throughout our day, we don't always breathe in and out on a count of 1, 2, 3.

I'm going to throw one more challenge at you by saying it's not enough to only time your pelvic floor exercises with your breath. If that's all you're doing, you're only getting about three- to four-second holds for the contraction piece. You also want the ability of your pelvic floor muscles to contract and relax as needed for longer and shorter periods of time and in times of inhales and breath holds, so they're ready for anything they may encounter.

So in the long run, it's great to challenge your pelvic floor to be able to continue squeezing as you breathe in and out and to squeeze your pelvic floor at intervals even faster than the way you breathe without hyperventilating!

Here's how to introduce quicks and longs to engage your fast- and slow-twitch muscle fibers.

1. **Quicks**: Squeeze and relax your pelvic floor in intervals of just one to two seconds for 10 repetitions. If you're used to timing your pelvic floor with your breath and find this change of pace difficult at first, try to talk out loud as you're doing these: "on, off" and "contract, relax," or try while having a conversation with a friend to ensure you aren't holding your breath or breathing too quickly. Remember, no one should be able to tell you're doing these.

2. **Longs**: Try to maintain a pelvic floor contraction longer than your typical exhale, but still continue to breathe in and out. Again, counting out loud to monitor your breath may be helpful. Shoot at first for a 10-second hold or even just five seconds. If that's where you start to feel your contraction, let go. Varying the intensity of your squeeze can change your endurance capability just like it would for strengthening any other muscle in the body. At a max contraction, it might only be realistic to hold for up to 10 seconds, while at a lower-level intensity, maybe with 25 percent effort you might be able to squeeze 30+ seconds. Whatever length you're trying to contract your pelvic floor for, make sure you let those muscles relax back down for equal or double the length of time before doing another rep. These take longer than the quicks, so maybe shoot for three to five reps total.

Adding quicks and longs in just a few times per week can be a great way to train your pelvic floor in a different way.

Because these don't necessarily come as natural with your daily movements, add them occasionally to habits such as brushing your teeth, taking your vitamins, checking emails, taking phone calls, or commercials during your favorite TV show or podcast.

Recap of Knowing Your Pelvic Floor:

1. Can you locate your pelvic floor muscles?

2. Are you able to contract, relax, and lengthen your pelvic floor muscles?

3. Do you plan to add a focus on lengthening your pelvic floor muscles (without breath-holding or straining) into your last few weeks of pregnancy?

4. Which exercises or daily movements of physical exertion do you plan to incorporate your exhale + contract and inhale + relax?

5. How might you fit in some quick, long, and varied-intensity pelvic floor exercises?

HABIT 3:
UNDERSTAND COMMON VERSUS NORMAL

Common: widespread, occurring frequently

Normal: occurring naturally; the healthy, natural state of the body

Just because something occurs frequently (common), doesn't mean it's the healthy, natural state (normal).

You are often given the advice to listen to your body. While I wholeheartedly agree and want you to be in tune with yourself, you know your body best. Knowing what to listen and look for can give you the confidence to go forward or slow down and ask for help.

This habit aims to prepare you to address issues that can occur anytime in life, especially during pregnancy. These issues are common (you're not alone!) but also not normal. You don't have to just live with them when someone says "oh, that just happens with pregnancy" or "it should just go away after pregnancy". The issues I will mention can be treated by a qualified pelvic floor physical therapist, other health care providers, or fitness professionals specifically trained in them.

Often addressing these things now will improve your quality of life throughout the rest of your pregnancy and your postpartum outcomes.

Normal versus common:

- Normal bladder habits versus leakage (urine, gas, and stool)
- Normal bowel habits versus constipation

- Normal pressure or gravity changes versus pelvic organ prolapse

- Normal stretching or separating of the abdominal muscles versus significant separation (diastasis recti abdominus) and symptoms to watch out for

- Normal changes in temporary aches and soreness versus persisting pain during pregnancy of any kind (low back, hips, pelvis, pubic bone, neck, wrists, etc.)

Bladder Norms versus Concerns

Are you peeing a lot?

Normal bladder habits for someone who isn't pregnant include voiding every two to four hours throughout the day. You typically feel your first urge to void when your bladder is about one-third full.

However, during pregnancy, you may be heading to the bathroom more often. Bladder habits in someone who's pregnant change first because of increased blood volume, thirst, and urine production and then later because of the actual pressure of the baby against your bladder.

Please don't restrict your water intake just because you're going more often.

If you're waking up frequently to void during the night and it's interfering with your sleep, consider:

1. Stop drinking fluids two hours before bed.

2. Elevate your feet at heart level or higher about two hours before bed for about 10 to 15 minutes and/or pumping your ankles up and down for a few minutes. If this feels okay to you, this may help you void one more time before bed by mimicking the lying-down position.

If you do notice changes in bowel or bladder habits that concern you, ask for help.

Common, *not* normal: leaking urine

Urinary leakage is also known as incontinence or peeing a little when you don't mean to.

Leaking during times of physical stress or exertion is called *stress urinary incontinence (or exertional incontinence)*. This may happen during:

- coughing, sneezing, laughing

- jumping (from the ground, on a trampoline, box jumps, jumping rope including double unders)

- exercising

- lifting

- running

- walking, stairs

- moving from sit to stand

- yelling

- vomiting

Leaking during times of strong urges is called *urge urinary incontinence*. This refers to the inability to make it to the bathroom in time.

Some triggers for urgency may include:

- Running water, seeing the bathroom, cold temperature, leaving the house or arriving home, key in the door, starting a workout.

Possible dietary triggers (irritation to the bladder lining): soda (diet and regular), coffee (decaf and regular), tea, juice, milk, chocolate—basically anything that is not water. This doesn't mean these drinks are bad. It just means that if you are experiencing urgency, you may want to consider the properties of what you're drinking such as caffeine, sugar, artificial sweeteners or flavors, carbonation, color, and acidity. Try minimizing or removing them from your diet to see if they are contributing to your urgency.

Alternating water between these drinks may also help decrease the irritation.

Mixed urinary incontinence means you're experiencing both stress and urge incontinence.

Leakage is *common* during pregnancy and postpartum. (Again, you are not alone!) Roughly one in three women will experience this in their lifetime, anywhere from childhood to old age. However, leakage is *not normal.*

Sometimes leakage is caused by an underactive pelvic floor and may require strength and coordination training to heal. Sometimes leakage is caused by an overactive pelvic floor and may require relaxation, stretching, manual work, and coordination strategies. Being examined by a pelvic floor physical therapist can be very helpful in determining the cause of your urinary incontinence and how to best treat it.

Healthy Bowels versus Irregular Bowels

Having a bowel movement at least three times a week to three times a day is considered normal, although most functional health providers consider at least once a day to be the norm. Your poop itself (yes, I'm going there!) should be smooth and easy to pass, not hard or watery. You shouldn't need to strain or hold your breath to poop.

Changes in bowel movements during pregnancy are common. You're not alone if you miss your daily dump, but you want to try to stay as regular as possible during this time.

Decreasing constipation can help you avoid the possibility of hemorrhoids, fissures, and buildup of pressure which could be painful and create or worsen prolapse and leakage.

It may be constipation if you are experiencing any of the following: going less than three times a week, straining, having hard stool, or difficulty passing stool.

Yes, that's right! I will say it again. You should not need to strain to have a bowel movement. There should be no breath-holding.

Tips for improving your bowel movement experience:

*Posture on the toilet: mimic a squat

Put your feet on a stool (typically six to nine inches of height) so that your knees are higher than your hips.

*Breathe: don't hold your breath!

Take a nice breath in, let your belly get big (don't forcefully push your belly out), and then as you exhale, try to gently relax and lengthen your pelvic floor without holding your breath or straining.

*Rest, meditate

Rest in the restroom. Don't rush. There are even guided meditations available to help improve your relaxation during this time.

Listen to when your body tells you it's ready to poop. Don't ignore it, even if the timing doesn't feel convenient to you. I don't mean you should sprint to the bathroom as soon as you feel this sensation, but honor what your body is saying, and head there sooner rather than later. Enjoy the pleasurable experience of being able to have a bowel movement. Don't let it be taboo or inconvenient. Own it.

Other tips for staying regular:

- Exercise.

- Keep up your fiber intake (veggies, fruits, flax seeds).

- Stay hydrated. Drink plenty of water.

- Take magnesium.

- Do your relaxation diaphragm breathing throughout your day.

Normal Gravity or Pressure Changes versus Pelvic Organ Prolapse

Normally, there will be tissue changes that occur overtime with gravity and pressure changes that come from growing a baby inside you, and then birthing that baby into this world.

When the pelvic floor (involving muscles and connective tissues) weakens, there's a possibility that the pelvic organs (bladder, uterus, and rectum) can descend.

Pelvic organ prolapse is when these organs descend to the point of creating a bulge in the vagina. A prolapse is common (up to 50 percent of women will experience this), but you might be able to do something about it if it's bothersome to you. Depending on the degree of this descent and your symptoms, you should consider conservative treatment with a pelvic floor PT.

Prolapse may feel like:

- Pelvic heaviness or fullness.

- A tampon is falling out.

- There's a bowling ball pressing down.

- Something is coming out of your vagina.

- You may actually see something like a bubble or bulge sticking out past the vaginal opening.

Prolapse is common and may be experienced during pregnancy or postpartum due to the pressure and weight of the baby on the pelvic region, weight gain, breath-holding, constipation, quality of connective tissues, and gravity. It becomes a problem if it's uncomfortable to you. It is also of concern if you see the bulge nearing or coming out of the opening of the vagina. The more you can do to strengthen and prevent excessive pressure on the pelvic floor (the connective tissue and muscles), the better.

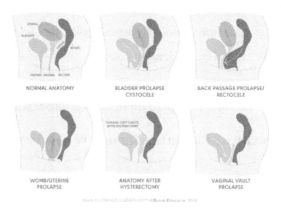

To prevent prolapse from worsening or to attempt to prevent it from occurring:

- Modify or avoid exercises and movements that cause any of the above symptoms.

- Avoid breath-holding or straining.

- Try to maintain regular bowel movements (decrease pressure).

- Perform your pelvic floor exercises correctly.

- Consider what role nutrition plays with the quality of your connective tissue.

- Get help from a professional trained in treating prolapse such as a pelvic floor physical therapist.

Normal Belly Stretch versus Diastasis Recti Abdominus (DRA)

As your baby grows inside you, your belly bump will expand. There is some degree of *normal* stretch and separation of abdominal muscles to give room for this expansion.

Diastasis recti abdominus (DRA) is when there becomes an excessive separation, greater than two finger widths of left and right rectus abdominis muscles (six-pack muscles) at the linea alba (the connective tissue between the two). The linea alba connective tissue runs from the sternum down towards the pubic bone. This area is meant to separate as a pregnant belly expands, so it is considered normal during pregnancy. And even when not pregnant, there is always some natural spacing between these muscles.

However, there are concerns for DRA when you are noticing doming, bulging, or coning while exercising or moving or you're feeling pain or discomfort in conjunction with these symptoms occurring.

There are some things that are more likely to make this gap worse than what is natural:

- Certain exercises based on your form, load, or duration
- Some postures depending on your form, load, or duration
- Breath-holding based on frequency or with load

During postpartum, this gap should slowly close in the following weeks and months. However, if you are concerned about this due to functional or aesthetic reasons, consider treatment with a physical therapist or fitness professional who specializes in DRA.

Pain: What Do We Know?

Pain is part of life. The experience of pain can be helpful in signaling to us to pay attention.

Pain at some point during pregnancy is common. Pain that continues to persist is not normal. If you're experiencing acute onset of pain, pay attention to what your body is telling you. Often, switching up positions, modifying your activity, moving around a bit, taking deep breaths, or using positive thoughts can help ease your discomfort.

If pain continues to bother you (don't just hope for it to disappear!), reach out to your health care provider for help.

Enjoy this time and don't let pain bother you or interfere with your daily activities.

It's better to try to improve your symptoms and optimize your health now than waiting until later.

Pain during pregnancy may include:

- neck pain
- carpal tunnel syndrome
- low back pain
- gluteal / butt / sciatic pain (one side or both)
- pelvic girdle pain (pain in pelvic region)
- pubic bone pain
- hip pain

Just because you're pregnant does not mean you need to suffer through this. There are lots of treatments. Depending on the cause (muscle, ligaments, joints, nervous system, or your brain's interpretation) and how long the pain has been persisting (recent versus ongoing) may affect which treatments you choose to pursue.

Most pain from tissues (muscle, ligaments, or joints) will resolve within three to six months as the body heals, but to help this process along, there are excellent treatment options for you to aid in the healing process, calm the nervous system, and give you strategies for coping.

Most pain that persists past the healing phase tends to be related to how the brain processes information and increased sensitivity of the nervous system.

In either case, these are some possible options you may consider exploring (some treatments are more for acute versus chronic pain, and some work great for both): physical therapy, breathing practices, dry needling, addressing your emotional and mental health, yoga, chiropractic, acupuncture, mindfulness or guided meditations, nutrition changes (inflammatory foods), learning about how pain works or pain education, massage/bodywork, and finding ways to better respond to stress.

Recap of Understanding Common versus Normal

1. Are you experiencing any common but not normal symptoms?

2. Do you have someone in your area you can reach out to if you do encounter these symptoms?

To find a pelvic floor PT near you, check out the locators at the end of this book in the Resources appendix.

HABIT 4:
EXERCISE IN A WAY THAT FEELS GOOD TO YOU

"Fall in love with your powerful body."

– Jessie Mundell, BPHE, MHK, P.Kin

Why?

Imagine you're going to compete in a major athletic event. Think ultramarathon, Ironman, CrossFit games, or whatever competition you think requires total beast mode.

What would you do? You train—at least if you want to improve your outcome during the event and your recovery after.

That's one of the main reasons that it's advised to continue or start exercising during pregnancy.

The major athletic event? Laboring and childbirth.

However, you're training for this with a body that's continuously changing and completely new to you. This will require training differently—both physically and mentally—than what you would in the above scenarios.

You are carrying a growing baby inside you, but not long from now, you're going to be carrying that baby all around with you, so you really want to train your body to have the stamina to endure it. However, you also do not want to do anything that could cause damage. Even if you have not been exercising up until now, it's still recommended to begin.

"Moving in ways that felt good to my pregnant body was crucial to recovering as well as I did. I loved suspension training, yoga, and walking while I was pregnant."

—Rachel Pufall, Breathe for Change wellness champion

Of course, always consult with your health care provider first as there may be some reasons unique to your case to back off or restrict exercise.

"I think it is important to emphasize that a woman's approach to exercise during pregnancy should be focused on optimizing health as compared with seeking specific fitness goals. Pregnancy is a time to learn to listen to your body. There is no reward for toughing out hard workouts during pregnancy. Rather, seek comfortable fitness challenges. Approaching fitness during pregnancy with honesty and self-awareness will be far more beneficial in the long run. It is still OK to work hard and sweat, but when your body tells you to slow down or stop, respect it. I find that many women push through running throughout their entire pregnancy (with pain and/or leakage) just to say they were able to do so. If running becomes uncomfortable, it is OK to walk. Even though you are a runner, walking when running hurts doesn't make you a wimp. It makes you smart."

—Meagan Peeters-Gebler, PT, DPT, CSCS, CMTPT

Dos and Don'ts

So what types of exercise should you do? To what intensity? How often?

"As a coach who works with a lot of high-level athletes who have only ever been told to listen to their body or do what they've always done, I've learned that they need so much more than that generic recommendation! They need to know what to listen for, why it matters, and how it will impact not just their fit pregnancy, but their recovery, symptom management, and overall long-term athletic performance. Having the ability to understand what to listen for and increased levels of self-awareness is the key for women navigating their fitness and life in general as it continually transitions."

—Brianna Battles, MS, CSCS

So, if someone tells you to listen to your body while making decisions, listen, look, and feel for:

- Peeing your pants (any leakage of urine, even a little bit during an exercise)

- Pain

- Breath-holding

- Pelvic heaviness, discomfort, or feeling like a tampon is falling out

- General discomfort or doubt about proceeding

- Separation, bulging, doming, or coning at the linea alba (the line between your right and left rectus abdominus—the six-pack abs). This is a sign of diastasis recti abdominus (DRA). Although normal to an extent during pregnancy, it is advised to modify or avoid activities worsening these symptoms.

- Difficulty breathing, fatigue, dizziness, or difficulty holding a conversation

- And any of the red flags listed at the beginning of this book

You should *never* push through the above symptoms. Some of these may sound common, but they are *not* normal. It's how your body is trying to tell you to stop, listen, and back off. Reach out to a provider or coach specializing in pre/postnatal fitness.

With that in mind, if you are not experiencing any of the above symptoms, weigh the risk and reward. What's your goal in doing this? Then proceed with *intention*. Many times there are ways to modify your activity so that you can stay active, but without the symptoms.

Find exercises that you enjoy! Find ways that feel good to move.

"Exercise isn't self-care if you are doing it as a form of punishment, damage control, or if you are doing it compulsively because it's the only tool you have to feel like yourself. Exercise is also not self-care if it hurts your body while doing it. If your body hurts for hours or days afterwards or if the effects compounded over time, it will eventually lead to injury or dysfunction in the future, nor is it self-care if you can't breathe comfortably and deeply while doing it. That's all. I just like to keep things straight since so many of us, especially in pregnancy and postpartum, find ourselves getting confused and often needing to redefine our relationship with movement and exercise during these transitionary times."

—Dr. Jaime Goldman, DPT, RYT, doula

In general, if it feels right to you, find ways to get your body moving about 30 minutes a day, five days a week. Put it on your calendar. Make it fun. Look forward to making the choice of when to exercise and when to rest.

How intense should it be? A lot of that depends on your activity level prior to pregnancy.

*If you're new to exercise, start out at low to moderate intensity.

*If you're already exercising, continue at the level you're at unless you're currently performing exercises that may compromise your pelvic floor or you are feeling symptoms mentioned above.

*If your body and mind tell you that it's time to slow down and start modifying, especially due to the experience of any of the above symptoms, please listen. Pregnancy is not the time to push through or set personal records.

Whenever you pick out exercises to do during pregnancy, my recommendation is do something you actually *enjoy* as well as what is *convenient* for you.

Everyone's pregnancy journey is different. Don't judge yourself on the person in the class next to you, your best friend, or your coworker. Sometimes you may be active longer, and sometimes you may have to modify or stop sooner.

Be intentional during this time. Why do you want to do or not do something? Remember that pregnancy is only temporary. What you choose to do and not do now will affect your postpartum recovery.

Set yourself up for success now and for your future self by finding the right activity level for you.

Exercise ideas

When trying to find what feels right to you, consider:

- walking
- hiking

- exercise in water: swimming, walking in water, water aerobics class

- strength training: lifting weights, using your bodyweight (squats, lunges, side planks)

- yoga

- dance

- stationary bike

- stretching: keep it gentle; don't push your limits while pregnant

- seeking out pregnancy-specific fitness classes (group or private setting)

If something starts to not feel right, here are some modifications to consider: changing your stride length, your pace, amount of weight, your posture or position, length of activity, intensity, and number of reps or sets.

For example, I love and highly recommend squats to everyone. However, I want you to perform them in a manner that feels right to you and your activity level. Some examples of modifying include using a countertop to hold onto while squatting. Being able to squat well will help with opening the pelvic cavity for childbirth. If at first you can't do a standing squat, try lying on your back and bringing your knees to your chest to improve your range of motion.

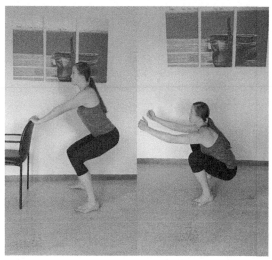

Just like with all exercise programs, it's good to warm up for a few minutes before you begin and make sure you cool down afterwards.

If you are unsure of where to begin with an exercise program, you need help modifying it, or you don't know what to listen or look for, please reach out to someone who has specialized training in working with pregnant women.

There are some activities you should avoid during pregnancy: high-risk activities such as contact sports, risk of balance or falling, skydiving, scuba diving, and high elevations. For more info, see ACOG guidelines (link in Resources appendix).

Recap on Exercise in a Way That Feels Good to You:

1. What is my mindset about exercising during pregnancy?

2. What types of ways do I enjoy moving?

3. Do I understand the signs and symptoms to listen and look for while exercising?

4. Do I have someone to ask if I need help modifying?

5. What are the benefits and risks to my choices in exercising during pregnancy?

HABIT 5:
GET SOME SLEEP

Sleep is important for a healthy lifestyle, especially with a growing baby inside you.

Make it a habit to prioritize quality sleep during this time.

Aim for seven to nine hours of sleep if possible.

Don't be afraid to take naps as needed. If you're able to squeeze it in, a 20-minute nap in the afternoon can be refreshing.

Why? Sleep is essential to healing and repair. Good sleep improves your muscles, blood vessels, heart, immune system, brain function, hormone balance, and more.

If you're having trouble sleeping, here are some ideas:

- Use pillows to help support you.
  - o Place pillow between your legs.
  - o Hug a pillow with your arms.
  - o Use a pillow for support behind your back.
  - o Use a pillow or towel under your belly while on your side.
- Stretch before bed.
- Convince your partner to give you a nice massage.
- Decrease screen time before bed.
- Set a specific bedtime.
- Make your room dark.

- If your mind is running crazy with thoughts before bed, record them into your phone or keep a notepad and pen near the bed.

- Only use your bed for sex and sleep.

- Exercise regularly and eat healthy.

- Practice breathing and mindfulness as you fall asleep.

- Talk to your baby about anything and everything (what you did today, your hopes and dreams, etc.).

What position should you sleep in? The one that feels most comfortable to you.

At some point, it will start to feel uncomfortable to lie on your stomach. Eventually, lying on your back might not feel great for long periods of time. Most women eventually transition to side-sleeping, and sleeping on your left side provides the best blood flow to the baby.

But don't fear if you wake up lying on your back or want to be there for part of your sleep. Most women report feeling the need to shift out of that position when it's time. If you start to feel uncomfortable in one position, switch to another.

Soak up the sleep now. Develop positive sleeping habits before the baby comes.

Recap on Getting Some Sleep:

1. How much sleep are you getting currently?

2. How is your quality of sleep?

3. Are you happy with your current habits as they pertain to sleep?

HABIT 6:
NOURISH YOUR BODY WITH FOOD AND DRINK THAT ENERGIZE

Nutrient-Dense Food

Nourishing your body during pregnancy is important not only for you, but also your growing baby. We should all eat quality nutrient-dense foods most of the time. If you've ever struggled with eating habits before, perhaps now you have a motivating factor of growing your little one that will help make these changes possible.

Here are basic suggestions for nutrition (from Michael Pollan's *Food Rules* book): "Eat food. Not too much. Mostly plants."

With a growing baby inside you, you should eat a bit more than your usual nutrient needs. However, a little doesn't mean you need to eat for two as in double what you're eating. Remember, a baby is small, so you'll actually burn more calories breastfeeding than growing a baby.

You only need about 300 more calories per day. Remember, not all calories are created equal. Try to aim for nutrient-dense food including quality vegetables, protein, and fat.

Listen to your body. It's about balance. Don't aim for perfection. Aim for learning what your body needs. If you're craving a very particular food like a donut, maybe your body could get its sugar craving from fructose in fruit. Not to say you can't have a donut. Indulge sometimes, but try to figure out what the craving might represent. What macronutrient or micronutrient does your body feel like it needs?

Try to add healthier sources of fat, protein, and carbohydrates, especially in the form of vegetables. Cooked leafy greens are a great choice. Get enough fiber and foods rich in folic acid, calcium, and other vitamins.

Overall, try to decrease spending your money and calories on things that won't nourish you as much: sugar, highly processed foods, refined carbohydrates, and empty calories.

You know your body best, though. Notice what gives you energy versus what slows you down and what gives you a restful sleep versus what gives you headaches.

Here are some healthy, nutrient-dense foods to consider incorporating:

- Carbohydrates: lots of vegetables including leafy greens, broccoli, sweet potatoes, squash, carrots, apples and berries

- Protein: beans, lentils, free-range eggs, grass-fed beef, free-range chicken

- Fats: avocados, seeds, nuts, and oil

"[Eat] plenty of leafy greens! My favorite way to enjoy leafy greens is via my lemony kale recipe. Though you can find the recipe in my book, it's a simple assembly of kale (curly or dino doesn't matter) lightly sautéed in cooking fat (butter is my favorite) until it's wilted down. Sprinkle with sea salt and fresh lemon juice and enjoy."

– Cassy Joy Garcia, NC

Nutrient-lacking and inflammatory foods to consider decreasing are highly processed foods, sugars, refined carbohydrates, low fat/fat-free/lite, additives, artificial sweeteners, colors, or preservatives.

Trying hard to change your food habits? Take pictures of your food before you eat it. Research shows this is helpful in reaching your goals because it increases your awareness.

Drink Plenty of Water

There are various recommendations as it pertains to water intake. Here are the top three:

- Drink 6 to 8 cups of water per day (8 oz. = 1 cup).

- Drink half your body weight in ounces of water per day. Example: you weigh 160 pounds ÷ 2 = drink 80 oz. of water daily.

- Drink water when you're thirsty.

Things that may affect your water intake are activity level, how much you sweat, and climate.

Notice that I'm specifically describing how much water versus how much fluids you should drink. All other forms of liquid and foods can contribute to some of your water intake. However, water is one of the best sources that you can get. Considering our bodies are made up of about 70 percent water, it's pretty important stuff.

Make sure you're drinking clean water. Test your tap water with a package of test strips. If needed, buy a filtration system to allow yourself to continue drinking tap water. If this option is available to you, it will save you money and the environment as opposed to buying water in plastic bottles.

Other forms of liquids sometimes have properties that could irritate your bladder or actually act as a diuretic, causing you to pee more.

Water is best spaced evenly throughout the day. Drink little sips at a time here and there to stay hydrated. Your body and bladder will appreciate the steady intake versus the flood-and-drought approach of chugging a lot and then withholding. Don't avoid drinking water because you're peeing a lot!

Ways to drink more water:

- Invest in a water bottle you love.

- Consider a fun color or stickers that make you excited to use it.

- Choose an insulated style to keep water at the temperature you prefer.

- Choose something that's easy to refill and wash.

- Notice if you prefer drinking from a cup with a lid, twist-off top, or straw.

- Use apps on your phone to track water intake.

Do you get bored with the taste? Add fresh fruit, lemon, or lime occasionally to mix it up.

Recap on Nourishing Your Body with Food and Drink That Energize

1. How are your eating and drinking habits?

2. Are you getting enough macronutrients and micronutrients and water to support you and the baby?

3. How can you improve your intake of nutrient-dense foods and water?

4. How can you decrease your intake of food and drink that are not nourishing you?

HABIT 7:
KNOW A BIT ABOUT POSTURE OR ALIGNMENT

Your body is adaptable, strong, and powerful.

For the most part, including pregnancy, we should be able to move and tolerate a variety of positions and movements. There isn't a specific posture or exercise that is bad in and of itself, but if performed repetitively, sustained for long hours of the day, or at high loads, there could be problems.

There comes a time where it's helpful to know a bit about posture or alignment changes that could help you. If you feel you can't get up and move as much as you want or certain positions or movements are beginning to bother you, pay attention.

Certain movements and postures may need to be modified briefly to ease discomfort, but usually, discomfort in a certain posture is your body's way of saying, Hey, I'd like to move.

Ideal posture doesn't really exist. However, having the knowledge and ability to change into postures that decrease stress on joints, ligaments, and muscles and to optimize breathing, pelvic floor muscle coordination, and other muscle recruitment strategies can be helpful.

We want to be able to move pain-free in all directions to function through life, but in general, here are some posture tips that can help optimize your body and have you feeling happier and healthier:

Guidelines:

- Ears over shoulders over hips over ankles

- Ribs stacked over your pelvis

- Pelvic bones parallel with pubic bones (pelvic tilt not too far forward or too far back—the ability to tuck and untuck tailbone and find the middle ground)

It's not about being able to stay in those positions all the time but rather the ability to get into them and use them to your advantage.

Posture begins to matter when you are in the same positions for long periods of time or you perform the same activity repetitively.

Posture Tips

Sitting

If you're someone who sits a lot, here are some ideas that might make your setup more comfortable:

- Sit with your butt all the way back in the chair so you can use the chair back as much as possible. Consider the use of a lumbar roll for more low back support.

- Adjust your seat to a height in which your feet can touch the ground, or use a stool under your feet if you can't adjust the height.

- If you enjoy crossing one leg over the other or sitting on top of one leg, consider varying the position of your legs. Switch somewhat evenly between right and left legs. Find a balance.

- If you have a computer or paperwork in front of you, try to get it at a height and distance that feel comfortable for your arms.

- Avoid having your computer too far away from you so that you aren't straining your eyes and rounding forward the entire time. If you reach your arm straight in front of you, the screen should not be farther than your fingertips.

- If you're operating on a laptop, consider a separate screen or keyboard so that you can have the screen at a comfortable height for your eyes (maybe raised up on books) and the keyboard at a comfortable height for your hands and wrists.

- Consider a way you can easily switch between sitting and standing at your desk. They have affordable options to super fancy options. A lot of times a large box or bin will do the trick too.

• Consider what you're sitting on. Sometimes switch to the floor, a deep squat, or sit on a Swiss ball to mix it up for a bit.

• Towels and pillows can work great for added comfort. Roll up a towel, place it horizontally along your low back curve, and/or place a rolled-up towel vertically along your upper back.

• Seat cushions can be helpful if you're getting some tailbone or low back pain.

More importantly, take breaks to get up and out of that chair and move.

Standing

We know sitting for too long is bad, but standing in one position for a long time isn't always great, either, especially if you're experiencing discomfort.

Are you always putting more weight on one leg? Do you jut out the right or left hip to the side? Are you able to stand symmetrically? Do you lean forward or backward? Again, it's great to have the ability to do all the above, but when repeated over and over, it has the possibility to cause some discomfort.

Here are some standing tips:

• If you like to unweight one leg while standing for longer periods of time, try putting your foot on a small stool to mix up your stance without compromising your hip jutting out to the side.

• Do you lock out your knees? Ideally, keep just a slight bend.

• How's your pelvis tilted? Do you tend to stand with your tailbone tucked way under or very untucked? Find a balance between the two the majority of the time.

• Footwear: Consider how different shoes change your standing alignment. The incline of high heels can cause you to shift forward like you're on a hill, but then your body has to work hard against that slope to keep you upright. Consider minimizing the height of your heels or time spent in heels.

Moving Around

Throughout life, you want the ability to bend, squat, twist, rotate, reach, and move in all kinds of directions. If any of these movements have caused you difficulty in the past or are starting to give you trouble, the key is to be intentional. Consider modifying your expectations, alignment, speed, load, and frequency to improve your comfort in these motions.

Here are some general tips:

Lifting: With heavier objects, move your body toward the object instead of reaching. Try to keep the object close to you. Attempt to keep the ribs stacked over the pelvis. Exhale on the lift. Try to pull back your shoulder blades and prevent your shoulders from rounding.

Bending: Find motion from your back, hips, pelvis, knees, and ankles. If you are bending to lift a heavy object from the floor, consider a squat or deadlift stance to optimize the use of your butt muscles (glutes) and legs. If this ever feels uncomfortable, vary your speed or depth to find what works for you. Make sure you don't hold your breath. Bend over and then exhale and recognize how much air you were trapping in your body.

Squats: Squat often! Squatting is a wonderful and underused movement pattern. If you have no reference for squatting, my first cues are "weight through your heels," "butt out," "chest up." But do whatever feels best to get you there comfortably. Hold onto a countertop or sturdy chair to work into a deep squat position if this isn't a normal part of your daily practice. This can help you with balance until you get stronger. Practicing squatting can help open your pelvis for labor and birth.

Walking: At times it may feel like you want to waddle, and perhaps that's because you've seen other women do it before, but as best as you can, try to stay as symmetrical. Attempt to keep a normal walking pattern. Just shorten your stride if needed. You've got this!

In or out of bed: Consider the log roll. Sit down on the side of your bed, and gently swing your legs up to the bed together in a bent position while you lower your upper half to the bed. This should result in you lying on your side. Do the reverse movement to get out of bed. This can help decrease pressure on your expanding belly and back.

While performing these movements, listen to what your body is telling you. If you're experiencing pain, leakage, abdominal separation and bulging, pelvic heaviness, or general discomfort, consider consulting with a professional who can help guide you through decisions for modifications of your daily movements.

Example: If you are experiencing pubic symphysis dysfunction (pain in pubic bone region), you may need to change your posture during movements such as getting in and out of the car, rolling over in bed, walking, and going up and down the stairs. Pretending the thighs are glued together and decreasing stride may be a helpful, temporary modification to decrease strain on the pubic bones. As my colleague Meagan says, "Live in a mini skirt with paparazzi everywhere."

Find a balance. Mix it up.

When trying to find the *ideal posture*, find a balance of what feels good and what is ideal. Make changes slowly and intentionally.

Any position for too long isn't great. Listen to when your body is simply asking you to change positions and mix it up!

Take breaks during repetitive tasks to rest or move in a different way.

If getting up from your desk or stepping away from your current tasks sounds unproductive, think again. Studies have shown that you actually increase your productivity if every half hour or so you get up to take a quick (even a five-minute) break to get out of your current position. So use that as a motivating factor if you are concerned about taking time for yourself to move.

Habit tips for changing positions:

- Consider setting a timer or finding an app that can remind you.

- Involve other coworkers or family members to encourage you and/or move with you.

- Do some pelvic tilts (rocking your pelvis forward and backward and tucking and untucking your tailbone). Move your pelvis in circles and figure eights. This is great for getting ready for labor and birth.

- Go for a walk.

- Stretch in a different position

- Post-it note that says *move* as a pop-up on your phone or computer.

Practice these postures now so that when the baby comes, it's easier to maintain these healthy habits.

Look ahead to what postures you may encounter postpartum, and come up with a game plan. Feeding the baby, lifting car seats, carrying the baby, and pushing a stroller are just some of the new positions and movements you will probably be encountering.

What types of positions and movements might be helpful for you to practice now? Do you have the right equipment or adjustments to fit your needs? Think ahead: a good tip for breastfeeding is to bring the baby to you, not you to the baby. Pillows can help with this posture.

Remember that you should be able to move in all different ways. It's only when you get stuck using the same dominant posture over and over again, repeated 24/7, that might get you into trouble.

Recap to Knowing a Bit about Posture or Alignment:

1. Are you able to get into a *good* posture, and how does it feel?

2. In what ways can you change up your sitting, standing, or moving postures to work smarter, not harder?

3. Are you changing positions and tasks to give your body what it needs?

HABIT 8:
PRACTICE SELF-CARE —
DON'T JUST CHECK IT OFF A TO-DO LIST

"Self-care during pregnancy isn't another item on your list of things to do or an added pressure or expectation in pursuit of *better* health. Self-care is an approach, a philosophy that guides your every moment. Self-care comes in many shapes and sizes. Maybe it includes rest, solitude, social connection, laughing, activity, time in nature, play, a difficult and honest conversation, a fun conversation, a warm hug, silence, effort, or service. But one consistent feature of self-care is self-compassion. Self-compassion includes having a clear nonjudgmental awareness of your needs and having the courage, kindness, and self-love to meet those needs, including asking for support when needed. Self-care and self-compassion are not selfish; rather, they are essential, so you have the inner resources available when required to care for and serve others, including the new life you are nurturing at this moment."

—Shelly Prosko, PT, PYT, C-IAYT

Self-care is important. It is essential. And it is a practice, not something to check off a to-do list.

Self-care can mean many things for different people. For some women, taking this time for themselves or finding ways to respond with self-compassion comes easy. For others, it is extremely difficult and takes practice.

Find a balance that works for you. This will be helpful for both physical and mental health.

Kindness and grace for yourself and stopping to just be in the present moment can fit into tiny pieces of your day. Some self-care is better than none. And just a little love can go a long way.

Improving the ways you respond to stress in your life can improve your sleep patterns and immune system. We can't control the things we cannot change, but we do have control over changing the way we respond to these stressors. This will build up resiliency and improve our self-care strategies.

Pick a mantra or affirmation and say it over and over again before bed, or post a note on your mirror that reminds you of *why* you're taking care of yourself and what motivates and inspires you.

Be an advocate for yourself every day, especially during pregnancy and your postpartum healing.

Having support now and for the fourth trimester (postpartum), especially in the first few weeks, is strongly recommended. Have a team to support you—people who you can call upon for help now and in your postpartum days ahead:

- Friends, family, partner
- Doula, birth coach
- Your health care providers
- Other supportive practitioners including those specifically trained to work with pregnant women: physical therapist, chiropractor, massage and bodywork therapists, acupuncturist
- Lactation consultants for breastfeeding help

Recap for Practicing Self-Care:

1. What does self-care mean to you?

2. What are the ways you can show compassion for yourself?

3. Do you feel confident being an advocate for yourself?

4. Do you have people on your team you can reach out to?

5. How do you feel you're able to respond to the stress (good and bad) that presents itself in life?

HABIT 9:
PREPARE FOR BIRTH AND RECOVERY

Being prepared for what's to come in labor, birth, and life after baby can be empowering.

It's also important to be ready for the unexpected. Go with the flow when your birth plan or postpartum plans can't always be achieved in the way you envisioned.

Here are some specific things that you can do to improve outcomes of labor, birthing and postpartum recovery:

- Take a birthing class.

- Decide how detailed (or not detailed) you want to be with your birth plan.

- Have a support system in place. Consider if a doula would be a good fit for you.

- Understand your options for labor and birthing positions and breathing and pushing patterns.

- Prep your perineum and pelvic floor for this big event.

But what about that last bullet point?

Perineal Massage

Typically, 35 weeks of pregnancy is a good time to start focusing on relaxing and lengthening the pelvic floor muscles and getting the vaginal opening used to pressure and stretch.

as a clock: 12:00 is up towards the clitoris and 6:00 down towards the anus.

2. With a clean finger (and potentially using some lubricant or oil), you or your partner can insert one finger about an inch into the vagina at the 6:00 position. Gently stretch downwards for up to a minute. You may want to start with 10 to 15 seconds and build up tolerance.

3. You can also gently make your way from the 6:00 position towards the 3:00 and 9:00 as if making a *U* for a few minutes.

4. You could enter two fingers and stretch outward and down at the same time.

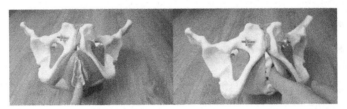

It should be noted that working on any older scar tissue (tears or episiotomies) in the perineum or cesarean scars is also a great idea. You can do this before getting pregnant again, while pregnant, or postpartum. A pelvic floor PT can help with this.

Breathing and Lengthening the Pelvic Floor (Preparing to Push)

*Practicing your lengthening of the pelvic floor muscles on the exhale ("belly big, belly hard" exercise from Chapter 2) can help prepare the pelvic floor to relax and let go to get ready for giving birth.

Consider positions that allow the greatest freedom the pelvis, sacrum, and spine as well as what feels comfortable to you.

Options to consider:

- hands and knees
- half-kneeling
- squatting
- lying on your side
- being in the water
- using a physioball

Packing Your Birthing Bag

Whether heading to a hospital, birth center, or having your baby at home, consider having the following on hand:

- Large chuck pads, incontinence pads, or diapers
- Underwear a size too big
- Pads that you can freeze to act as an ice pack on your perineum
- Compression shorts that go up to your ribs or a tight-fitting belly band or tank top

After birth, it's not necessary, but it can be very helpful to add compression to your pelvic floor and abdominal region as the swelling decreases and the muscles start to come back to their normal length.

I typically recommend that you use the compression support of your choice during the day of your first week. Take it off at night to give your body a break.

In the second week, start to decrease the use to times you're up and moving more (roughly 50 percent of the day).

By the third and fourth weeks, wean off the compression and feel more of your own core strength beginning to activate. Wear 25 percent of the time during periods of more activity.

From day one postpartum and for the next few weeks, it's important to rest and let your body heal. Consider staying off your feet for the first few weeks. Ask for help if this recommendation feels far-fetched. Spend time in bed or on the couch healing. Aim for rest and ask for help to achieve this in the early days. Perform gentle breathing exercises. When you do need to exert yourself (getting up from sitting, rolling over in bed, lifting baby), exhale to decrease pressure on the pelvic floor, and make it easier to move. Set very small goals to slowly increase your activity tolerance. This portion of exploring your new life with a baby should be taken seriously to allow your body to heal. Be intentional with your mind and body.

Six Weeks Is Not a Magic Number

Continue to listen to your body postpartum for the signs and symptoms mentioned throughout this book. There may be days you feel ready and restored to get back out there, and there may be days and weeks where your body screams rest. Your mindset and choices in movement should be intentional with an emphasis on breathing and pelvic floor strategies. Do what you can to find a balance, and continue with self-care.

When you reach the time of the six-week checkup, speak up if things don't feel right and if you have questions about how to function in this new body and life of yours. Six weeks is not a magic number, and I encourage you to ask for help if you have concerns. And maybe you feel OK at six weeks, but symptoms arise later at six months. Speak up then. It's not too late.

I would highly encourage you to ask for a referral to a pelvic PT for postpartum rehab that can address things that are sometimes overlooked. This is a standard practice in France and other countries where their rates of pelvic floor dysfunction are significantly less in postpartum women who complete pelvic floor PT.

1. Do you understand how to perform perineal stretching starting at 35 weeks of pregnancy?

2. Do you feel empowered about your breathing for birthing?

3. Do you feel like you have options for your labor and birthing positions?

4. Do you understand the importance of healing postpartum and taking it slow as well as asking for help if things don't feel right?

Final Words

You were made to do this. You are a strong, beautiful, powerful woman, but know that if something doesn't feel right to you, you don't just have to live with it.

There are people and resources out there to help you reach your best pregnancy ever.

Well, are you ready to rock your pregnancy? How do you plan to make these healthy habits stick?

Practical advice:

- Pick just one to two things to focus on at a time.
- Don't try to change everything at once.
- Figure out which habits resonate with you.
- Which do you feel motivated to practice?
- Use your free bonus checklist found at the end of this book or pdf version at *http://jentorborg.com/Pregnancy-Checklist*

When figuring out what to do or not to do during pregnancy, trust that voice inside your head, and ask yourself why. Weigh the risk versus reward.

Also, think about times in your life when you made a positive habit stick or when you were able to ditch a negative habit.

Why did it work?

What tools help you follow through on goals?

Do any of these resonate with you?

- Accountability through support groups locally or online

- Reading up on the research behind some of these recommendations

- Scheduling it into your planner

- Setting reminders or goals on an app

- Writing out motivating notes on why you want to make the change

- Announcing it to others

To your best pregnancy ever!

You're ready to leave your imaginary pelvic floor physical therapy BFF chat and begin adding in the habits you wish to your daily life.

You can reach out to me if you have questions or need help finding a pelvic floor PT near you at *jentorborg.com*.

The second book in the pelvic floor physical therapy series covers many topics for postpartum health including:

- pelvic floor rehab (general core strength, how to work on leakage or prolapse, and DRA)

- what to do about scar tissue (cesarean, episiotomy, tearing)

- more posture tips for life with baby

- return to activity, including running and higher-level sports

- return to sex

I wish you the best of luck on this adventure.

PERSONAL EXPERIENCE

I wrote this book based on my professional experience prior to experiencing pregnancy and childbirth myself. I got pregnant shortly after I published *Your Best Pregnancy Ever* and *Your Best Body after Baby*. Here I will include my blog posts about my own experience including my outdoor home birth story. All blog posts were originally published on the Vagina Whisperer website (*https://www.thevagwhisperer.com/*) and can still be found there.

- Tips for First Trimester
- Tips for Second Trimester
- Tips for Third Trimester
- Jen's Outdoor Home Birth

TIPS FOR FIRST TRIMESTER

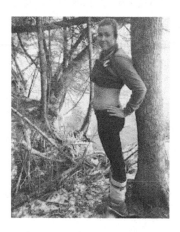

1ST TRIMESTER ADVICE BEFORE BEING PREGNANT AND NOW WITH REAL-LIFE EXPERIENCE.

I found out in October 2018 that I was pregnant with my first! After working with many women during pregnancy and postpartum for over five years, I was stoked to start the journey myself and be better able to see if my pregnancy advice was legit. I'm going to share with you the advice I gave to moms in their first trimester: what I talked about in the clinic, to my friends and in my book, Your Best Pregnancy Ever . And then I'll include what this advice turned out to be like for me in real life at the start of my pregnancy.

STAY ACTIVE.

Find ways to workout and move your body that feel good to you: yes to this! So many studies and my clinical experience show that staying active during pregnancy can help mama feel better during pregnancy and improver her postpartum recovery as well as baby developing. During my first trimester, I was hit with fatigue and nausea. I found that working out actually made me feel better (or some days at least not worse), so I sucked it up and got some sort of intentional movement. Some days the fatigue or nausea hit me harder and I skipped the workout and rested. I soaked in the sleep when I could. I learned that I still highly value physical activity for pregnant mamas including myself, but that it was also important to listen to my body and find a balance between pushing past some of the tired days and other days enjoying rest. I enjoyed moving through walks with my dogs, yoga, step class, strength training, short runs and adventurous hikes.

WORK ON RELAXATION TECHNIQUES.

That includes deep breathing and self-care strategies to honor your body, mind and soul during this time. Real life: big yes! Especially on those rest days, but even on the active ones, I attempted to better listen to my body. I was careful about what I said 'yes' so that I didn't overbook my schedule. I worked on diaphragmatic breathing at home, at work, while driving. I journaled, listened to good music and took some baths.

START CONNECTING WITH YOUR PELVIC FLOOR.

It's important to know how to contract, relax and lengthen your pelvic floor muscles while understanding how to coordinate this with your breath, movement and everyday life. I was lucky enough to get "only" the constant nausea for weeks, but not the actual vomiting. In preparation for my pelvic floor being able to handle morning sickness should it strike, I definitely upped my pelvic floor exercise game. Find a balance between contracting and relaxing both in isolation throughout the day (sitting, standing, lying down) as well as with movements (getting up from a chair, lifting, bending, exercise routine). If you're not sure how to contract or relax your pelvic floor, or have any symptoms of pelvic floor dysfunction (urine leakage, pelvic pain, pelvic heaviness, etc.), please reach out to a pelvic floor PT near you or check out our virtual sessions. I love how many mamas in their first trimester have been reaching out to us for prevention or early treatment feedback

EAT NUTRITIOUS FOODS AND STAY HYDRATED.

Yes, but... it was harder than I thought. My very first wave of nausea hit with onions. I was so revolted. As someone who's never been a picky eater and literally always wants to eat food, this has been one of the most bizarre experiences for me so far. There were a few weeks where I really did not feel interested in veggies and craved bland foods like bread and crackers. I tried to sneak some veggies in where I could and tried to add quality sources of fat and protein to the bland carb choices I craved when possible. But it didn't come easy to me and I humbled myself during this experience. Lucky for me as the first trimester came to an end and I transitioned to the second trimester, I felt I was able to eat most foods again and could start picking nutritious foods that energized me, gave me quality sources of protein, fiber, fats and carbs. I will say that staying hydrated with water was really helpful to my nausea and energy levels. So that part felt right. I just kept refilling my klean kanteen every chance I could get!

Also, I've been using a squatty potty for years and continue to highly recommend getting a stool of some kind in early pregnancy if you haven't already. This can really help improve bowel movements by better relaxing the pelvic floor muscles that wrap around the rectum when you get your knees higher than your hips. And breathe during your bowel movement!

ENVISION YOUR PREGNANCY/BIRTH EXPERIENCE.

It's never too early to begin to build up a team around you - interview midwives, OB/GYNS, find a pelvic floor PT near you, a chiropractor, massage therapist, acupuncturist, a mental health counselor, prenatal yoga, prenatal fitness instructors, etc. You want to have options in mind for if/when you need them or to contact for wellness and prevention. You do not need to build up your whole team right away, but it's nice to have options and give yourself time to ask friends, professionals, social media, etc. for recommendations and to set up interviews.

I interviewed my midwife team once during the end of my first trimester to get to know them, their services and my insurance/financial options, but waited to set up my first intake appointment until I started my second trimester. There's no right or wrong way. Just do your research and see what options feel best to you.

Although I haven't set up other visits yet I have a person in mind for most of the other professionals I listed as suggestions. I live in a rural area, and for me about half my potential team is local and the other half virtual.

TIPS FOR SECOND TRIMESTER

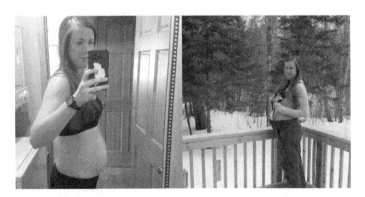

REFLECTIONS ON MY 2ND TRIMESTER: NEW FOUND ENERGY, LEG CRAMPS, PELVIC FLOOR EXERCISES AND MORE.

Well, I'm 32 weeks pregnant and finally taking the time to write about trimester #2. At first pregnancy felt like it was going sooooo slowly (maybe because I told people when I was only ~6 weeks pregnant). Now it's definitely flying by quicker. The first few weeks into the second trimester didn't feel much different than the first. I was still nauseous and tired most of the time, but trying to stay active and rested as much as possible. But then, like magic, a few weeks into trimester two, I felt awesome. Well, maybe not totally awesome, but better than how I had been feeling and more like myself again. I had more energy. I was no longer feeling nauseous. I could start eating veggies again without getting grossed out. I know for some people the nausea, morning sickness, fatigue, and other not so fun symptoms can last throughout the whole pregnancy, so I was relieved that I was able to get a break.

EXERCISE!

I used my new found energy to go on daily walks and keep up with movements such as squats and lunges both in the strength sense and as a stretching version. For strength, I do squats and lunges in repetitions (example: 10 reps x 3 sets with or without added weights). For stretching, I do a supported deep squat by holding onto a countertop to get low for a pelvic opening position. For stretching lunges, I did a hip flexor stretch (target the muscles in the front of my hip/thigh) in a standing lunge or kneeling lunge. I did have a little intermittent low back pain and lower abdominal discomfort during this time as my belly started to visibly expand. I used a belly band support occasionally during the day to help ease this discomfort.

YOUR PELVIC HEALTH BOOK

I also used this burst of energy to decide to write and publish my third book, *Your Pelvic Health Book* during the second trimester. Yes, I'm a little crazy. I heard this time in pregnancy it's great to take a nice vacation or get some big projects done you might not get to after baby. For me it was to write a book. This required time and effort, and I recognized my need for quality nourishment, staying hydrated with water, taking breaks to get outside, walking in fresh air and getting as much sleep as possible between writing, editing and marketing.

LEG CRAMPS

As the final weeks of my second trimester came to a close and I was transitioning to the third trimester of pregnancy, I started to get some leg cramps. Darn charley horses had me squirming and catching my breath during the night. To help remedy this, every night before bed I began stretching my calf muscles which was the main place I felt the cramps. I also used magnesium lotion to rub into these muscles. And I upped my water intake, and I wore compression socks. Within a night or two of prioritizing tackling leg cramps, things felt much better.

PELVIC HEALTH IMPORTANCE

The other thing I continue to focus on throughout this pregnancy is, of course, my pelvic health. On a daily basis I did pelvic floor contractions AND relaxations throughout my work day while sitting or standing. I also added these in while exercising, walking and with exertion like lifting a heavy dog food bag. If you've been following the Vagina Whisperer or any pelvic PTs you probably know by now that urinary leakage is common, but not normal. So far, no leakage for me. I contract my pelvic floor with coughing and sneezing and avoid straining by exhaling with bowel movements or heavy lifting. I find ways to be aware of my pelvic floor subconsciously and purposefully with exertion. It's become second nature now. It also helps that I'm teaching people about their pelvic floor on a daily basis and therefore getting plenty of reminders.

I'm so grateful for the knowledge and resources I have as a pelvic floor PT to help support me during my pregnancy. If you have any aches, pains, leakage, or pregnancy concerns that you feel might be helped by a pelvic PT feel free to reach out to us for virtual pelvic wellness sessions.

JEN'S 3RD TRIMESTER

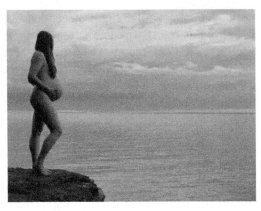

Looking back on my third trimester, (I'm now 7 weeks postpartum but finally getting a chance to write out my thoughts) I'm going to share with you a bit about what I loved, what I disliked, what I think helped, and my thoughts during week 40 and 41.

WHAT I LOVED ABOUT THE THIRD TRIMESTER:

Watching my belly grow. I was amazed at what my body was capable of.

Feeling the baby move - kick, punch, wiggle, dance and hiccup. It was weird and awesome at the same time.

My ability to stay active. As an able-bodied woman who loves being active and outdoors, I was very thankful to still go on hikes and daily walks with my big belly bump without too much difficulty.

WHAT I WASN'T FOND OF:

Heartburn... ugh. I got this a lot and it seemed pretty unpredictable. Chewing gum and drinking lots of water may have helped me some.

Shortness of breath and slower walking speed.

Fatigue and tiredness. Lots of naps and early bedtimes. I was thankful lots of sleep was an option for me!

Sleeping positions got uncomfortable even with all the pillows for support. I missed being able to lie on my stomach.

Sciatica - I only had a few brief experiences of this. Luckily I was able to self-treat and have a coworker help me out. I used stretching, manual trigger point release with a ball and my hand, foam rolling and dry needling.

THINGS THAT HELPED ME ALONG THE WAY:

Being proactive in attempting to decrease the amount of swelling:
Compression socks. I wore Sockwell's during my work days or days I was going to be on my feet and more active.
Legs up the wall, legs elevated and ankle pumps.
Walking!

Moving my body in ways that felt good:
Cat/cow, Child's pose and sitting on a physio ball doing pelvic tilts and circles.
I continued to walk a lot usually still hitting 10,000+ steps a day as long as it felt good. This was usually walks

outdoors, walks with my pups and walks with friends which equated to some mental self care, too!

Staying hydrated:
>8+ cups a water a day felt good to me.

Staying positive:
>I listened to a pregnancy and birthing affirmation CD when driving.
>
>I journaled on what I envisioned and hoped for my labor and birth experience while still remaining open and calm about childbirth being variable.

Pelvic Floor exercises!
>I continued to do pelvic floor exercises (kegels, but more than that...) with breathing, in isolated positions, with movements and all sorts of variety.
>
>I focused on contraction, relaxation, and lengthening with breathing to prepare for labor and pushing. **If you're not sure what I'm talking about, check out my pelvic floor physical therapy book series, Your Best Pregnancy Ever or schedule an online session via the button below.**

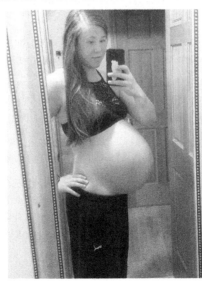

Final Notes

If you find yourself nearing your due date and are feeling antsy, here were my thoughts during that time…

40 weeks pregnant was a time of gratitude and reflection. "I'm grateful… For the Big Lake, the Gitche Gumee, that called us to Chequamegon Bay. For the friends and healers that have shown me so many possibilities exist for pregnancy and birth. For the way I have felt confident in making this pregnancy journey my own: a mix of research, intuition and the support of others, especially my amazing husband. For allowing nature to teach me so much during this time: patience, presence, transitions, being open and flexible. I'm excited for what will come next. I'm excited to meet our little one. But today I'm grateful for what this experience has been so far."

41 weeks pregnant: "I've told many friends and clients over the years the stats, as well as, some version of the saying "baby will come when baby is ready." A "due date" is simply an estimate of 40 weeks gestation, not necessarily when baby is expected to arrive. First time pregnant people average 41 weeks + 1-4 days before they go into labor naturally. Meaning the other half will go beyond that. Despite my knowledge, as well as, trust in my body and in my baby, there are moments in these last days of pregnancy that are challenging me physically and emotionally. But with challenge comes growth and so I lean into it. My midwives at the Ashland Birth Center are amazing and they have been a tremendous help to my mental health throughout this pregnancy. This week, they sent me a beautiful article describing this "place of in between" and it's truly been a help for me to read these words and continue to accept this unknown. Below is an excerpt.

> *"The last days of pregnancy — sometimes stretching to agonizing weeks — are a distinct place, time, event, stage. It is a time of in between. Neither here nor there. Your old self and your new self, balanced on the edge of a pregnancy. One foot in your old world, one foot in a new world."*

I made it through the 3rd trimester. If you enjoyed this, please check out my birth story (at home and outdoors with midwives!). If you're pregnant and looking for ways to decrease or prevent pain (back, hips, pelvis, pubic bones, etc.), leakage, pelvic heaviness or have other questions about pregnancy and postpartum reach out to us for an online consult.

JEN'S OUTDOOR HOME BIRTH

I learned that birth outcomes can truly improve if a person is in an environment they feel comfortable and respected in whether that be at home, at a birth center or at a hospital. Whether that be with midwives, doulas, OBGYNS, family practice docs, just yourself, your family or anything in between. I realize that privilege (racial, financial, education, health status, etc.) can play a large role in what choices someone has available to them, but my hope is that someday we can all have the quality birthing experiences we desire and deserve.

I envisioned a birth that felt right for me and my family. My goals for birth came about through a mix of research and intuition. I practiced affirmations and mindfulness exercises daily to visualize my dream birth (including reading through this website and changing the narrative slightly to make it my own) . And it happened. My birthing experience was challenging and hard, but also beautiful.

On Saturday, July 6 I started pre-labor contractions. My husband, myself and our dogs went for an early morning 3 mile hike (I'm grateful I was able to stay so active during pregnancy) and I was feeling some mild contractions every 10 minutes that lasted about 20-30 seconds. After arriving home from the hike we did a lot of nesting: cleaning the whole house, mowing the lawn, preparing the birthing space (I was planning a home birth). At one point in the evening my contractions started to get more intense and painful. They were close together (~2-5 min), but still very short in length (~20 sec), so I took a warm bath which helped slow down the intensity and frequency. I was really hoping to get some sleep that night to prepare for a possible birth in the early morning. However, I continued these pre-labor contractions throughout the night. The contractions were too frequent and too intense to get any sleep, but was able to use this time to adjust to what was happening with my body all while my doggie doulas offered cuddles.

Sunday, July 7. I believe my active labor began around 2 a.m. At that time the contractions were becoming more intense and I headed to the shower. The warm water helped calm me and allow me to process what was happening. Around 4 a.m. I decided to send out a text to my team of midwives telling them that I was confident I'd been at 5-1-1 (every 5 minutes 1 minute long contraction for over 1 hour). I let them know I was still doing okay solo, but that I was probably going to call one of them within the hour if labor kept progressing. By 4:45 a.m. I knew I was ready to have others join me and I made the call. I told one of my midwives I was ready to have her come check my progress, but no need to rush. Then I went to wake up my husband and tell him he should probably call into work because "I think this baby is coming today." :)

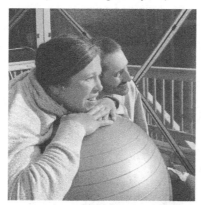

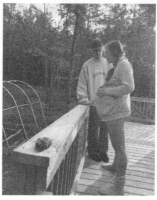

By 5:30 a.m. my first midwife arrived. She watched me through a contraction or two and then with my request and consent checked my cervix. She let me know that I was fully effaced and that I was dilated to 4cm but quickly opened to 6cm while she was checking. After her confirmation that this was really happening, my contractions continued to intensify. I felt a release in my body and a connection with my baby that we were really ready to do this. I started to be more vocal and really go into the contractions. I felt

wild and powerful. I kept my eyes closed for a lot of my labor and just went inside my body/experience. I labored on the couch for a bit on my hands and knees and then sitting on the toilet. Around 6:30 a.m. my second midwife arrived and shortly after I wanted to be outside. We headed to the deck as the sun was rising. Around 7:30 a.m. the student midwives (two of them) also arrived. My whole midwife team also happens to be dear friends of mine and I'm so thankful I had them surrounding me during this experience. Throughout labor, my husband was always near me holding my hand or putting an arm around me as I needed it. My dogs were also a big part of my comfort, giving me little licks or letting me pet them which brought me peace.

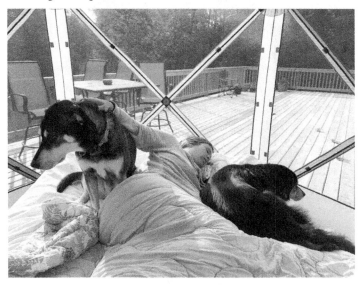

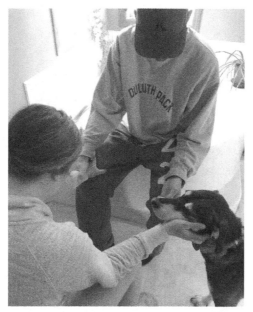

Around 9:30 a.m. I felt the urge for the first push. The pushing phase was the hardest part of labor for me, both mentally and physically. *Full disclosure, it was really hard for me to put my professional mind aside and connect with my body's need for breathing versus breath holding while pushing.* Also, my water still had not broken and I could feel a resistance from that. I tried pushing for a while outside and slowly took off layers as the sun continued to climb. I began to get too hot and we decided to move the bed over to the shade, which was the original area we envisioned for our baby to be born. I tried pushing there for a bit, but was still having difficulty. At one point I let out a cry for my waters to be broken, as I knew intuitively I wanted this relief of pressure to be able to progress. My midwife broke the water bag and I felt a huge relief. I then decided that it would be best to connect with pushing on the toilet, so back inside we went. I squeezed my husband's hands hard and gritted my teeth against our hand hold. I held my breath more than I ever expected to, but it's what I felt like I needed to do at the time. During contractions prior to pushing, I felt I could exhale or be vocal during the sensations, but during pushing I felt the need to breath hold and use that pressure to push baby out (this isn't what I typically teach, however, I do always recommend following what your body is telling you). After some more progressing and pushing in on the toilet, I was able to feel my baby's head start to come to the opening.

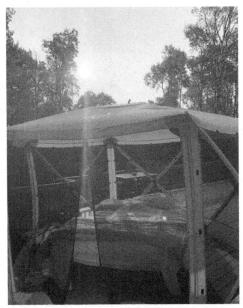

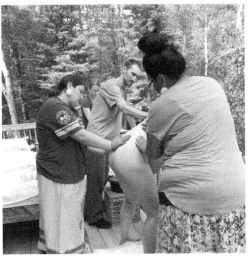

We really wanted our baby to be born outside, so my husband held me in a slow dance embrace and we walked back out to the deck where we initially envisioned birthing at. As we got outside I stood along the railing looking out to the trees. I pushed a few more times. I felt my baby's head. My husband felt the baby's head. And then I gathered all the remaining energy and strength I could and I pushed my baby out into my husband's hands. It was 11:02 a.m. I didn't plan to birth in a standing position, but once again I listened to my body.

My husband caught our baby and then helped bring baby into my arms. There baby was, earth-side. We lied down together in the bed and cuddled baby to us. The dogs took turns meeting baby. It was around then that I looked down to see the sex of our baby. An awesome surprise. I really thought I was about to see a penis, but instead I saw a vulva.

I was still having some strong cramping and shaking in my legs, so the midwives helped deliver the placenta while we were lying down. And then it was done. What an amazing birth. It felt so awesome to give birth to our baby outdoors at our home surrounded by trees. Elements that felt comfortable to us.

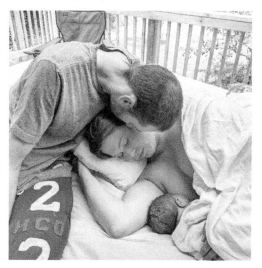

After birth, we headed inside to bed where the midwives tucked us in and made us breakfast in bed, which was amazing. They did a few newborn tests while we all lay in the bed and bonded.

Baby weighed 8 pounds 10 ounces and was 21 inches long. We named her Rowan after the rowan tree and for our love for nature. On day two, we gave her the middle name Sofia after the Greek word for wisdom.

And that's my birthing story. It was amazing and I'm so thankful it went so smoothly. There are so many choices available to us in our birthing process. And there's no right or wrong way. There's no medal for doing birth a certain way. And sometimes your birth doesn't go the way you want. If you're struggling with your birth not going the way you wanted, I encourage you to reach out to others, share your story and heal when you're ready.

Do I recommend others birth at home like I did? Only if it's something that you want. Do I recommend some people go to a birth center or hospitals or have epidurals or have a water-birth or even recommend some have elective cesareans? Yes, absolutely. It's all about being informed as much as you can, or as much as you want to, and then making a choice that feels right for you and your family. You don't owe an explanation to anyone. You do you. And best of luck!!

YOUR BEST PREGNANCY CHECKLIST

Healthy Habits to empower you in pregnancy, birth & recovery	I'm rockin' it!	I want to work on it...	Here's what I plan to try (example: 5 breaths before bed, walk with a friend on Tuesdays)
#1: Embrace breathing			
Am I avoiding breath holds? Am I breathing while I'm moving?			
Am I using relaxation breaths throughout my day?			
#2: Know your pelvic floor			
Do I know where my pelvic floor is?			
Can I feel my pelvic floor muscles contract, relax & lengthen?			
Am I using my pelvic floor muscles with movements?			
Do I plan to focus on length-ening my pelvic floor muscles - without breath holding - starting at 35 weeks gestation to prepare for labor & birth?			
#3: Understand common vs normal			
Do I have someone I can reach out to if I experience any of the following: leakage, constipation, prolapse, diasta-sis recti, pain?			

#4: Exercise in a way that feels good!			
Do I have ways that I enjoy exercising? Am I taking time to exercise?			
Do I know how to listen to my body and modify exercise if needed?			
#5: Get some sleep			
Am I getting 7-9 hours of quality sleep?			
#6: Nourish my body			
Am I eating nutrient dense foods that nourish me & my baby?			
Am I drinking enough water to support myself & baby?			
#7: Posture & alignment			
Do I vary postures so that I move in different ways throughout the day?			
#8 Practice self-care			
Am I showing compassion for myself?			
Do I have ways to positively respond to stress?			
#9: Prepare for birth & recovery			
Am I up for perineal massage/ stretching starting at 35 weeks?			

Do I feel empowered about breathing & possible positions during labor & birth?			
Do I understand the importance of healing postpartum & taking it slow?			

DID YOU ENJOY THIS BOOK?

It would be really great if you would leave a review on Amazon so others can find out if this book would be helpful to them.

I truly appreciate you taking your time to do that.

ACKNOWLEDGEMENTS

Using my platform to empower women would not be possible if it weren't for:

- The contributions of those that paved the way: Julie Wiebe, Tracy Sher, Amy Stein, Shelly Prosko, and many more!

- The mentorship of Meagan Peeters-Gebler

- The support of Orthopedic & Spine Therapy

- The UW-La Crosse PT program and especially my partner in all things pelvic and obstetric, Kelly Diehl

- All of my wonderful clients I've had the pleasure of working with

- And the support of my family and friends, especially my awesome husband, Alex!

RESOURCES

To find a PT near you:

- American Physical Therapy Association Section on Women's Health PT locator: http://pt.womenshealthapta.org/

- Herman & Wallace | Pelvic Rehabilitation Institute: https://pelvicrehab.com/

- Pelvic Guru: Find a Pelvic Health Professional: https://pelvicguru.com/2016/02/13/find-a-pelvic-health-professional/

Links to those providing quotes and support:

Introduction

- Casie Danenhauer, DPT

    o Enlighten PT http://www.casiedpt.com/

Know Your Pelvic Floor

- Tracy Sher, MPT, CSCS

    o Pelvic Guru www.pelvicguru.com

    o Sher Pelvic Health www.sherpelvic.com

- Burrell Education

    o www.burrelleducation.com

- Amy Stein, DPT, BCB-PMD

    o Heal Pelvic Pain http://www.healpelvicpain.com

    o Beyond Basics Physical Therapy http://www.beyondbasicsphysicaltherapy.com/

- Julie Wiebe, PT

    o Julie Wiebe PT www.juliewiebept.com

o Online courses
http://www.juliewiebept.com/products/online-courses/

o The diaphragm pelvic floor piston demo:
https://www.youtube.com/watch?v=mLFfZfm7O7c

o The diaphragm and the internal pressure system:
https://www.youtube.com/watch?v=cW9mwfy-6-I

- Pelvic Model

  o http://esp-models.co.uk/composite-pelvispelvic-floor

Understand Common versus Normal

- Burrell Education

  o www.burrelleducation.com

Exercise in a Way That Feels Good to You

- Jessie Mundell, BPHE, MHK, P.Kin

  o www.jessiemundell.com

- Rachel Pufall

  o Breathe for Change wellness champion
  www.breatheforchange.com

  o Yoga instructor at Ignite Fitness
  https://www.ignitefitnessstudio.com/

- Meagan Peeters-Gebler, PT, DPT, CSCS, CMTPT

  o Orthopedic & Spine Therapy, Appleton, WI
  http://www.ostpt.com/therapists/meagan-peeters-gebler/

- Brianna Battles, MS, CSCS

  o Everyday Battles: Strength and Conditioning
  www.briannabattles.com

- Dr. Jaime Goldman, DPT, RYT, Doula

  o Luna Physical Therapy
  www.lunaphysicaltherapy.com

- ACOG guidelines for Exercise
https://www.acog.org/Patients/FAQs/Exercise-During-Pregnancy

Nourish Your Body with Food and Drink That Energize

- Michael Pollan: *Food Rules*
https://michaelpollan.com/books/food-rules/

- Cassy Joy Garcia, NC

    o Fed and Fit http://fedandfit.com

Practice Self-Care

- Shelly Prosko, PT, PYT, C-IAYT

    o Physioyoga: www.physioyoga.ca

    o Full blog post on self-care: http://physioyoga.ca/self-care-the-dark-side

    o More resources: http://physioyoga.ca/pelvic-floor-galore-resources-for-creating-pelvic-floor-health-through-yoga

    o Video practices on Vimeo:
    https://vimeo.com/ondemand/pelvicfloorhealth

    o 10% discount code for Vimeo video practices:

    ClientDiscount10

ABOUT THE AUTHOR

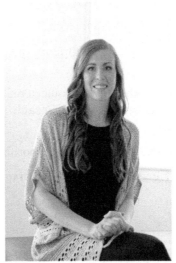

Photo credit: Kelsey Lindsey

My name is Jen Torborg. I'm a licensed physical therapist with a passion for pelvic floor physical therapy. My goal is to empower you on your journey to understanding your body and mind better during pregnancy and postpartum and while dealing with pelvic, bladder, bowel, and sexual dysfunction. I am the author of three books in the Pelvic Floor Physical Therapy Series: *Your Best Pregnancy Ever*, *Your Best Body after Baby*, and *Your Pelvic Health Book*.

I received my doctorate of physical therapy (DPT) from University of Wisconsin-La Crosse. I have my Certificate of Achievement in Pelvic Health Physical Therapy (CAPP-Pelvic) and Certificate of Achievement in Pregnancy/Postpartum Physical Therapy (CAPP-OB) from the American Physical Therapy Association (APTA) Section on Women's Health (SoWH). I often incorporate dry needling in my practice, and I am a certified myofascial trigger point therapist (CMTPT) through Myopain Seminars.

I strive to provide a positive, comfortable environment to treat clients in Ashland, Wisconsin at St. Luke's Chequamegon Clinic. I also work with clients virtually through pelvic wellness sessions at The Vagina Whisperer. I look forward to educating my patients about their body and how they can take control of their health.

Outside of my career, I have a love for the woods and the water. I live in the Chequamegon Bay region of Lake Superior. Home is being surrounded by trees and trails with the love of my life, Alex, our daughter, Rowan, and our two dogs, George and Lucy. I enjoy being in nature, which gives me a sense of calm and restores me. I love minimizing and tidying. And I'm inspired by a beautiful sunrise.

Made in the USA
Monee, IL
15 March 2022

92497066R00056